Dentistry and how it's damaging your health

Stefan Cairns

BALBOA.PRESS

A DIVISION OF HAY HOUSE

Balboa Press books may be ordered through booksellers or by contacting:

Balboa Press
A Division of Hay House
1663 Liberty Drive
Bloomington, IN 47403
www.balboapress.co.uk
UK TFN: 0800 0148647 (Toll Free inside the UK)
UK Local: (02) 0369 56325 (+44 20 3695 6325 from outside the UK)

Print information available on the last page.

ISBN: 978-1-9822-8774-0 (sc)
ISBN: 978-1-9822-8773-3 (e)

Library of Congress Control Number: 2023919711

Balboa Press rev. date: 10/16/2023

FOREWORD

I met Stefan about three and a half years ago at his very first Alliance Meeting of Huggins trained dentists. He was a newbie. I had just given a presentation to the group on Oxygen/Ozone therapy. He was full of questions and enthusiasm. We sat together at dinner that night. He asked so many questions that evening about dentistry. This guy, I thought, really wants to know this information about the science of mercury fillings, root canals, infections and the immune system of the human body. As a Huggins trained dentist and practicing now for over 31 years, I have had many conversations with Stefan and witnessed the logarithmic learning he has achieved. Stefan learned from 17,000 patients, their problems, their symptoms, their failures, and their successes.

Stefan quickly became a leader and advisor in the Huggins organization. Now, I may not agree with Dr. Huggins' method 100%, I feel that his protocols are some of the best in the dental field for dental revisions and building up the immune system to achieve a healthy body and mind. He has been revered by many patients and dentists throughout the world. Stefan has followed Dr. Huggins obsessively for those years, not only through shadowing him but also "walking the talk". He has gone through an extensive dental revision and detox and has gained health and wellness, and experience through it. God only knows what kind of mess Stefan would be in physically and mentally if the forces had not brought him to the Huggins Center.

Stefan is knowledgeable and experienced. You don't work with that many people 24/7 and not gain the ability to counsel patients affectively. This guy knows a lot! Trust him (as I do) with his knowledge and let him lead you on a path of wellness!

It is an honor to write this forward for Stefan Cairns.

John A. Rothchild, DDS, FAGD, MAGD, DAAPM, NMD,

Doctor of Integrative Medicine, Dentistry and Naturopathy

Assistant Professor Emeritus, Capital University School of Integrative Medicine

Former Dean, School of Integrative Biological Dental Medicine

Dedicated to

Billie Patterson

Loved and missed by all who knew him

God bless you Billie

I will start this e-book with a statement of fact, I am not a doctor/medical professional/PhD or scientist, I am however a man who worked as the Client Service Director for Dr. Hal Huggins for three and a half years.

Dr. Huggins treated more than 3000 patients over a 40 year period, a large percentage of them had what was generally perceived to be an incurable disease, and his success rate in treating these patients was 86% meaning 86% had a significant reduction in symptoms.

I have read every book written on the subject of health by Dr. Huggins, plus several by Dr Thomas Levy and other very knowledgeable professionals.

During my time with Dr Huggins I talked and helped more than17, 000 clients.

This book will cover a variety of areas relating to your health, so often the mouth or specifically your teeth is overlooked as the source of your health problems.

Your mouth is the always open store, the 7/11 of your body; you breathe, eat and drink through it, it's the most convenient way of getting unhealthy bacteria into that much-overlooked precious temple... Your body.

The comments I make in this book are all based on the teaching from Dr. Huggins that I was blessed to receive, in addition to the books authored by him and/or Dr Thomas Levy, confirmation of all data can be found in the list of books in the glossary at the end of this book.

CONTENTS

DETOXIFICATION

During my time working for Dr. Huggins I constantly came across clients wanting to go through some form of detoxification or chelation, my first question was to ask why?. The standard response was "***to remove the heavy metals from my body***" it has been proven that these come primarily from the amalgam fillings placed in the teeth over the years.

I can understand why this would be a strong desire especially as the person had been experiencing one form of health problem or another and often this had been the case for several years.

I would then ask if they still had amalgam fillings in their teeth, if the answer was yes then I'd explain that there was no point in using one of the many forms of detox or chelation at this time.

To do this was a little like trying to dry yourself while still in the shower…yes that does sound a little silly but that is what they would be doing.

The amalgam was, and is the greatest source of mercury released into the body, every time you chew, brush your teeth or drink hot drinks you stimulate the release of methyl mercury which is 100 times more toxic than mercury, mercury is the most toxic non radioactive substance on earth.

So, detoxification is simply not a viable option until the amalgams have been removed.

Now back to the subject of detoxification, I will cover this assuming that there are no amalgams in your teeth.

We've all seen and heard the many claims that a particular product will remove all heavy metals from your body in two days, or one week or a month. All you have to do is drink this unction or potion twice a day or take this pill with all meals or whatever…

Some, I'm sure will have some positive effect's however, most don't…mercury is not an element that actually wants to leave the body once it has found somewhere to live. The problem is that blood tests in the main will not show mercury in the blood, it's devious, it hides, and I liken it to the Taliban or some other terrorist organization. They wouldn't wander the streets of NY holding a banner claiming to kill all the American infidels. No, they would take a job and pretend to be an active member of the community.

Ok so what do I mean by this, your blood cells all carry an identifier like a number plate on a car, this is called a Major Histocompatibily Complex (MHC). This is unique to every person; your immune system constantly looks for "non self" cells, when found the alarm bells are sounded

The first line of defense is Globulin, part of the total protein in your body. Globulin will rush in to attack the invader, but sadly, mercury is indestructible to anything the body can throw at it so all that happens is the globulin is rendered totally ineffective and the mercury now has a hiding place.

So, when you have your blood tested by those wonderful people telling you that their product is "***the best thing since sliced bread***", mercury doesn't show up, and "**wow**, this amazing product has done its job...no it hasn't, it's just that the mercury is hiding.

To my knowledge there is only one way of actually finding the level of mercury in one's body, this test is done by a wonderful company called "Quicksliver Scientific" in Lafayette, Colorado run by Chris Shade, PhD.

This is a methyl and inorganic mercury test, and as far as I know, Dr Shade is the only one in the country doing this. At the beginning of 2011 the cost was $250.00.

There are several tests that can be done in addition to the methyl mercury test that will help, please spend some time at their web site.

Dr Shade is a wonderful man and can be contacted:

303 531 0861

Info@quicksilverscientific.com

The test is done by Quicksilver Scientific but you still need pay to have the blood draw, this is done through a lab such as LabCorp or Quest Diagnostics, you'll need to do your own research here because the blood draw can vary from $35 to $100. At the end of the day it's just a blood draw and should be on the lower end of the scale.

Probably the easiest and least traumatic way of detoxifying is to use the C-flush method which is basically using Vitamin C or Sodium Ascorbate powder, when doing this you should always ensure you have the following ingredients:

Sodium Ascorbate powder

Probiotic capsules/tablets/drink

Activated charcoal capsules

Electrolyte drink

Or you can call Huggins Applied Healing and buy the C-Flush package which includes all the above. 1 800 948 4638

This process is best started on a Saturday if you work during the week; this is to allow a day of rest following the C-flush.

The program is done over a 7 week period, week one you start by taking one gram of sodium ascorbate powder (roughly a level teaspoon) in 2 oz's of water, mix thoroughly and swallow.

This is done every 20 minutes until the onset of diarrhea, it typically takes 8 or 9 grams to induce diarrhea, and once the diarrhea starts it will normally continue for a couple of hours. Do not take any more sodium ascorbate powder that day. If however diarrhea hasn't started by the fifteenth gram you should stop and try again the next day.

You should drink the electrolyte drink to replace those lost during the elimination; I found that taking two activated charcoal caps a few hours after the diarrhea has stopped will also help in preventing an unexpected reoccurrence.

Now I said this is done over a 7 week period so here are the specific instructions:

Week 1.

One gram of sodium ascorbate powder in 2 oz's of water every 20 minutes until diarrhea starts, continue to eat normally during the day. Take two charcoal capsules several hours after the diarrhea has stopped, also take the electrolyte drink and the Probiotic.

The following day should be a day of rest and recuperation because you will feel rather drained and a little tired.

Week 2.

Repeat the process as per week one.

Week 3.

Repeat the process as per week one.

Week 4, 5 and 6.

Eat normally; take no sodium ascorbate powder.

Week 7.

Repeat process for week one.

This is the least traumatic way of detoxifying and one that is recommended by Dr. Huggins.

When I first joined Dr. Huggins, I wanted to try the C Flush so I would have firsthand experience and be able to honestly relate my findings to the clients I talked to each day. So during the first seven weeks I used this method of detoxifying and found it quite helpful and very easy to do.

If you've had your amalgam fillings removed and there is a very specific procedure to do this which I will cover later in the book under the heading Amalgam fillings. A couple of weeks later you can start the detoxification through a vitamin c flush or another very useful and effective product is IMD made by **Quicksilver Scientific**.

IMD is **Intestinal Metal Detox** which comes in a powder or 100mg capsule form, the contact information is listed earlier in this e-book.

I personally used this product with very positive effects for 18 months, during this time I had no negative side effects.

In fact when I first met Dr. Shade in 2008, we discussed my health problems, I had been diagnosed with multiple sclerosis (MS) in 2004 so he suggested I use the IMD and gave me a three month supply.

I had recently gone through a Total Dental Revision with the wonderful Dr. Blanche Grube so exercising wasn't an option for me initially; however after a three month wait which was very difficult for me I was able to start to gently exercise.

During the first week of using IMD I was taking it in the morning after eating breakfast, Dr. Shade had suggested I take it on an empty stomach but that just didn't work for me as it gave me an upset stomach. However after I started taking it an hour after my food in the morning I started noticing very positive results.

Before I started on IMD I tried exercising but it was still very difficult for me, an exercise called a squat thrust, starting in a push up position then jumping your legs forward and backwards.

I managed 6 pathetic squat thrusts, I was embarrassed at my feeble attempts, however a week after using IMD I was able to do 20 squat thrusts, then 30 minutes later I did another 20.

Over the next month it improved to sets of 60 three times in the evening, meaning I did 180 each day.

As far as I know the product costs around $130 for a 10 week supply, taking one per day, 5 days on then 2 off.

Another method recommended by Dr. Huggins would be a hot bath or/and a far infra red sauna, now if both are used, they should not be done both on the same day, I'll explain the reasons why.

Firstly the hot bath is probably the easier and cheaper method than far infra red sauna; it is only the cost of a bath of hot water and some Epsom salts.

Run a bath of hot water, but not too hot, the temperature should be only as hot as you feel comfortable stepping in without burning your feet or making that "*ah*" sound. Pour a cup of Epsom salts into the running water, swish it around to mix the salts effectively into the water.

Make sure you have a ***bath sheet,*** a large bath towel, lower yourself into the bath and pull the bath sheet around you in the water.

Stay in the bath no longer than you feel comfortable, this would vary between people, so I suggest no longer than 15 minutes. Then stand up and shower yourself off, do not wipe the water off yourself first as all this will do is push the excreted mercury back into your skin.

You can do this three times per week.

If you have a Far Infra Red Sauna, only use this on the days you are not taking the bath, alternate between the two, only use the sauna three times per week. This is because your body can only detox at a certain speed. Think of it this way, if you had a wide mouthed funnel, you can pile whatever you want funneled as quick as you like, however the other end is only a narrow tube. So, it will come out at a much slower rate, meaning the material you are trying to detox from will overflow which will cause you to feel sick or at least very unwell.

I'm talking from experience here, while going through a detox after my dental revision and feeling very good about myself. I *"overdosed"* on my detox. Sad because I'm very good at giving advice but it seems not too good at taking my own, is that a man thing? So I learnt the hard way, and want you to benefit from my own silly mistakes.

Over the years I regularly spoke to people who asked about chlorella, my opinion is different from Dr. Huggins, he tells people to stay away from this product because it comes from the ocean. In his opinion anything from the ocean and that includes all forms of sea food/fish/plankton etc is contaminated with mercury.

I have the utmost respect for Dr. Huggins and the amazing work he has done over the years and I'm not saying that he is wrong, at the end of the day I am just me, Stefan Cairns, I'm not a doctor/PhD/Scientist .just someone that worked for him for three and a half years.

However I did a great deal of research and I believe your mind should be like a parachute, it doesn't work unless it's open. With this attitude I put a great deal of faith in Dr. Joseph Mercola who has the biggest natural health website in the world.

Dr. Mercola talks very positively about chlorella products and the effectiveness in heavy metal removal.

www.drmercola.com

AMALGAM FILLINGS

To this day there are still millions of amalgam fillings every year being placed into the teeth of unsuspecting people in the US alone, even though the rest of the world or at least Europe has outlawed these killers. I'm not being overly dramatic when I describe them as killers because long term that's just what they are.

An Amalgam filling is an amalgamation of dissimilar metals; prior to 1976 they consisted of 52% mercury, zinc, copper, tin and maybe 8-10% silver. So when the dentist tells you he is going to put a silver filling in your tooth/teeth quite frankly it's a blatant lie…Its mercury primarily. Mercury is the most toxic non radioactive substance on earth; it gets worse because every time you brush your teeth, drink hot drinks or chew you stimulate the release of methyl mercury which is 100 times more toxic.

After 1976 the filling was "updated or upgraded" to the high copper amalgam filling, this is equal parts of mercury, copper and silver. Even though there is less mercury it stimulates the release of methyl mercury 50 times faster than the original.

The most sensitive parts of your body are the insides of your cheeks and under your tongue, so you can imagine where the elemental mercury goes…..yes into your body and your blood stream.

The blood consists of red and white cells; the white is essentially your immune system, its primary role is to protect you from invaders.

The red is broken down into roughly 30 components; one of which is hemoglobin which has 4 ports on each cell to carry oxygen….oxyhemeglobin.

Mercury attaches to one, two, three or even all four ports so is now transported around your body, it doesn't want to wander aimlessly, it wants to find somewhere nice to live, like a filter organ, your liver, kidneys, heart or brain. Once resident there it will prevent the organ from doing its job efficiently and "***hey presto you have symptoms***".

I have always found it quite ridiculous to think that the wonderful trusted community of general practitioners (GP's) insists on treating symptoms and not the cause of the problem. So you see your doctor, are then told to take a medicine/drug and the chances are, you will be on medication for the rest of your life…***nice.***

In 2008/9 a school in Lakewood, Colorado was closed and 600 pupils were sent home, why, you ask, well there had been a spillage of a hazardous material so the HAZMAT team were called in. Now I'm sure you are thinking that there had been a large amount of a radioactive material spilled, well you would be right in thinking that way. In fact it was a mercury thermometer that had been broken.

Now if 600 kids were sent home because a very minimal amount or mercury was spilled on the floor why oh why is it considered safe to allow **larger** amount as an amalgam filling to be placed into uninformed, unsuspecting people? Thousands of times every day of the year.

This is interesting; did you know that the ADA actually holds the patent on amalgam fillings? So those wonderful, considerate people are actually being paid every time an amalgam is placed. It's no wonder they refuse to acknowledge the dangers in these hideous little killers. When it's eventually accepted worldwide that amalgams are killing people and the ADA have always known this then there will be an even bigger law suit than there was with the tobacco industry.

Let's move back to amalgam fillings, because of the amalgamation of dissimilar metals, your saliva and the warm environment of your mouth, these fillings have all the basic requirements to be little batteries. They emit a signal, an electrical signal, negative or positive, high or low. **Perhaps fillings could be better described electrically by calling them capacitors. Capacitors, like the flash portion of a flash camera, build up a charge over a**

period of time, and then discharge much of their stored current in an instant This is measured in micro amps'; having an electrical signal requires them to be removed in a very specific sequence. There is only one way of identifying that signal and that is to use a RITA meter, this device that was created by Dr. Huggins. It's similar to an ammeter or amalgameter but there is very significant difference and that is the RITA meter measures the peak of the signal and stays at that point. This is crucial because the fillings need to be removed sequentially, starting with the highest negative; after that one has been removed the remainder of fillings in that quadrant can be removed.

Now it becomes a little confusing as the remaining fillings starting with the next highest negative are to be removed following the guide in the previous paragraph.

However, the dentist needs to check all the fillings in the mouth; they are marked on a chart by his assistant. If, after the first quadrant has been done the next highest negative filling is on the other side of the head crossing the midline, draw an imaginary line down your head splitting your eyes, down your nose and thru your lips, then there has to be a 48hr gap between removals unless the dentist is using **Conscious sedation**. The most popular or commonly used is **Versed** which is similar to Valium. If conscious sedation is used then after the first highest negative filling is replaced the sequence doesn't apply.

When Dr. Huggins noted this several decades ago he found that if this protocol is not adhered to, then 63% of patients develop an autoimmune disease, not necessarily immediately but it is likely to happen at some point.

There is almost a conspiracy here between the dentists that have done the honest research and found that Huggins work is real, and the powers that be like the American Dental Association (ADA) plus their cronies like Device Watch or Quack watch. These people will spread malicious misinformation about the pioneering work of Dr. Huggins and Dr. Weston Price before him. I have spoken with my clients and uninformed dentists who truly believe there is nothing wrong with an amalgam filling. This is because of the misinformation being spread by the ADA…

I'm sure you'll be thinking "I'll just go and see my local holistic or biological dentist, because he or she will do it right" well the sad thing is that NO, they won't. There are lots and lots of very competent, experienced dentists, some biological, some holistic and they will tell you that they are very experienced in the removal of amalgam fillings. They have done it thousands of times, "*so just come see me and I will take care of you*".

Again I can't emphasize this strongly enough, biological, holistic, means nothing when it comes to the only safe methods of removing and replacing amalgams.

A Rita meter should be used to identify the correct sequence of removal; the dentist should use a rubber dam, oxygen, water, powerful suction and a Negative Ion Generator to ensure a clear channel over the dental chair. Some dentists will also use some form of suction device to clear the air immediately around the patient.

I'd like to ask this of the dentist's that profess to be able to competently remove amalgams, "***when you've removed the amalgams the wrong way, do any of the patients ever come back in six months or a year and tell you they now have MS or one of the other incurable diseases.***" No, they don't because the patient didn't realize it was the dentistry that caused the problem, Dentist's are living in a dream world! I believe that the pharmaceutical industry are responsible for the millions of people suffering from ill health these days however I also believe the dentist's are guilty and in some ways even more so.

There is only one safe way to remove amalgams, and that is to follow the protocol laid out by Dr. Huggins as listed above, over the years I have talked with thousands of clients all stating that they had had their amalgams removed the correct way, most, not all but most would tell me that they had seen a Huggins trained dentist, to which I would ask for the name of the dentist and the city or state they were in. Some people wouldn't tell me the name, why, I just don't know; maybe they thought they would get the dentist into trouble.

For those that did tell me the name, it would often be a name I'd never heard before. What their dentist probably meant was that they attended a two hour seminar and shook Dr. Huggins hand, so in their mind they had been trained. The client would try to justify the dentist's work, this I just couldn't understand because the client would be suffering from health problems and often serious health problems which are likely to have been caused or at least instigated by dentistry.

Dr. Huggins holds trainings twice each year or at least he did, this would be a three day training program held in Colorado Springs, normally in March and October although that could vary by a month either side depending on when the IAOMT were holding their semiannual seminars. **My recommendation is to find a Huggins trained dentist, this can be done by calling Huggins Applied healing on 1 866 948 4638.**

At the end of this book I have listed the dentists that were considered to be an elite group of Huggins trained dentists including the city and phone numbers.

One particular dentist in my opinion stands head and shoulders above the others; this is because of her experience and unequalled skills. Dr. Blanche Grube has followed Dr. Huggins work closer than anyone else for twenty years.

Her passion, compassion, skills, experience and dedication surpass all others, I will not go into detail about a health challenge she experienced because I feel it best coming from her. Needless to say she has been there, done that and has the T-shirt and video when it comes to health issues.

BIO COMPATIBLE MATERIALS

When amalgams are replaced by the dentist, and hopefully a dentist that has been through the official training with Dr. Huggins, he or she should only place filling material back into your teeth that is bio compatible with your blood. There are lots of good filling materials available to dentists, some good because the supplier/manufacturer is providing this product at a good price or a special deal for the dentist. But that doesn't mean it's good for you the patient, what is good for you is a material that is bio compatible with your body which is essentially one that will not have any adverse reactions when placed into your teeth.

How is this done? Well there are several ways but in my opinion there is one that is more accurate than the others.

You will often be told about "muscle testing" or kinesiology, this is where the dentist will have you hold a particular material in one hand then ask you questions while pressing down on the opposite arm which is extended out.

I don't really have a great deal of confidence in this method, I'm sure there are some very qualified practitioners in this field but I'm a little uncomfortable with this method, I just feel that it can fluctuate if you or the dentist had a bad night last night.

So from my experience and having researched the various ways of identifying which material is going to be safe in your teeth/body I always come back to the bio compatibility test.

This is done by calling Bio Comp Labs is Colorado Springs, 1 800 331 2303.

They will send you a kit which you take to a lab such as LabCorp or Quest Diagnostics; the kit includes instructions for the lab and the necessary vials.

Your blood is drawn then spun on a centrifuge to separate the blood from the serum. The serum is then put into a small vial which is put into a larger vial then into a polystyrene box and finally into a cardboard box. This is very important and part of the kit that is sent to you. You should then overnight it back to Bio Comp Labs, this should never be done on a Friday as it will wait in a truck for two days until Bio Comp Labs open on the Monday morning. So ideally have the blood draw first thing on a Monday morning on an empty stomach, fast for at least 10 hours, then overnight it to Bio Comp.

They will basically run tests with your blood serum against the 96 materials that dentists have the ability to use plus another 3000 materials to identify what material your body will tolerate. Please note that I said your body…not some other person's body just yours. So they will specifically tell the dentist what is safe for you, a material that your blood is saying is acceptable for you. Now this is a more scientific method but even this cannot be 100% accurate, it's close but the human body is a fragile/delicate and unpredictable thing.

Bio Comp Labs will then mail or email a 62 page document to the dentist so you can feel confident he or she knows which product is safe for you. The dentist can pre order this product if they don't have in on their shelves.

The kit is free to you and will be sent upon your order which you can do over the phone or online.

The cost of the test was $275 in April 2011, but remember you'll have to pay for the blood draw with whatever lab you chose to use.

There is another company that professes to do this test accurately, however I don't have a great deal of confidence in them. I know at one time they didn't test for aluminum which I'm sure most people realize is a major contaminant. With this in mind I would only use Bio Comp Labs.

Now I know some people will complain about the price, this is your choice, is your life worth $275?

Don't have it done and take the risk that the dentist will somehow manage to place a filling material into your teeth that your blood will not have an adverse reaction to. You'll often be told that a particular material is good for most people, this statement may be true, **but then again are you most people?**

I've probably talked with more than 5,000 people who thought the same way and regretted it because they came down with Chronic Fatigue or Fibromyalgia or another of the many diseases waiting to find an unsuspecting body to thrive in.

TOXICITY OF DENTISTRY

Quite often the source of a health challenge would be right in front of you, or as Dr Huggins would say...Right under your nose. Yes in your mouth, or more specifically, your teeth.

After working with Dr Huggins for more than three years and reading some very notable and knowledgeable authors like Dr. Hal Huggins, Dr. Thomas E Levy, Dr. George Meinig and of course the original master, Dr. Weston A Price. I feel confident in my understanding and experience; **however *I will never recommend, or prescribe a product or procedure based on you telling me of your illness or disease, because I'm not qualified to do that*.** However I will share my experience and knowledge and if you have results similar to the thousands of others I've talked with then I'm sure you'll be happy.

As mentioned earlier, your blood can tell you so much about what is happening in your body, At Huggins Applied Healing we would look at a blood test, this test was quite comprehensive and would indicate several things to us. The test would be a Blood profile and CBC with a manual differential.

Now I have to make that statement very clear, myself or Carolyn being the most experienced in the company at the time were not the ones making assessments, judgments or recommendations on what was happening in a client's blood. No, this was only done by a computer program which had been created based on Dr. Huggins work. This was the Huggins Recovery Program or as it was later known, The Assist Program.

However, Carolyn and I would look at the program results and over the years became very knowledgeable and experienced in understanding what was happening in the blood.

The Blood profile and CBC with manual differential consisted of 35 components, ranging from Calcium and Phosphorus right down to the red and white cells plus the five components of each.

As I mentioned earlier the blood is very complex, not just some red stuff that flows through your veins.

Components of the blood such as Bilirubin, AST, ALT and LDH will provide an indication as to what is happening in your liver, every component in the blood is affected by the others, so correcting one area will affect another area. So when you see your doctor who tells you are a little run down and suggests taking an iron tonic please understand that although it will increase the red blood cells it won't necessarily improve the effectiveness to carry oxygen (oxyhemeglobin) to the areas of your body crying out for help.

This is why the Recovery program is so effective; it will look at all areas of your blood and address each of the deficiencies or surpluses as they relate to each other.

The Assist program is available from Dr. Huggins office, the cost as of April 2011 was $765.00. As with any program based on your specific blood you will have to pay for the blood draw which can vary from lab to lab. My recommendation would be to join Life Extension; the cost of joining is around $75.00 per annum. You can then have the blood test at a very reasonable price,

The number to contact Life Extension on is 1-800 208 3444

The next paragraph is directly from the work of Dr. Huggins, I felt that this would be a valuable addition to this book.

When a healthy body is challenged with a toxin or antigen, what happens to the white blood cells? They increase in order to defend the body and reestablish its homeostasis. If the toxins do not go away, what does the healthy body do? It increases the defense team. That means that it brings on additional white blood cells.. In the case of mercury escaping from a filling, the questions becomes how many white blood cells does it take to remove all the mercury coming out of it? The answer should be billions and billions, if it were indeed possible. The real answer is that white blood cells cannot remove all the mercury coming from the filling, but they fight anyway. Is it possible that the really super healthy body constantly increases the number of white cells thinking that it can eventually win the battle by overcoming the enemy by sheer number? Outsiders, that is doctors not living within the body or really understanding its dilemma, come up with a name to describe the event. The label is leukemia, which describes the conditions of massive battle. The treatment is to kill off those white cells in order to reestablish homeostasis. What is missing is understandings that the white blood cells are just behaving in response to their job description in trying to defend your life. This is not a slam toward our system, just a suggestion of one more way to look at a problem that has found very little help over the past three decades. Maybe it is an accommodation for survival.

Taken from "The Mechanics of Toxicity", by Dr. Hal Huggins.

I have added this to show and justify dealing with the cause of the problem not just the symptom which is traditionally what is done by the average GP, and doctors treating patients in hospitals.

ROOT CANALS

A ROOT CANAL IS OFTEN RECOMMENDED to a patient that has been having a minor problem with a tooth, slight pain or discomfort but then again it could be that you have had a fall and knocked the tooth so that it's moving in the socket.

You experience this problem and see the dentist as your savior, someone that is going to relieve the pain and make it comfortable for you to eat again, *what a nice person*.

Well I suppose this paragraph is going to upset a lot of people, patients and dentists alike. A root canal is a bad thing, in fact it's the worst thing a woman can have, it's bad for men but the absolute worst thing a woman can have.

I'll explain that in more depth a little later but now I'll tell you why the dentist is recommending the root canal. You think it's because it's best for you, well no it's not. but it is the best thing for the dentist.

Firstly it's a very lucrative business, it probably takes the dentist an hour, and I'm being generous here, so an hour's work relates to $1,000 to $1,500, good pay for an hour's work.

Secondly the ADA had a requirement for dentists to place 40 million root canals each year, well that's what it was at the end of 2007. In their infinite wisdom they changed that in 2008 to 60 million by 2012.

So American dentists have a quota to fill, yes they have so many to do each month, in fact the staff are encouraged to promote root canals to patients.

I remember in 2008 I was talking to a woman that had called in for information; she told me that she had recently moved to a new state. She called a dentist in the town she had moved to, the receptionist asked why she was calling and was told why she needed to see a dentist. *"A slight pain in my front tooth"*, the receptionist replied with *"sounds like you need a root canal"*. Now this is the recommendation from a receptionist on the end of a phone line not a dentist looking into her mouth.

Fortunately the woman did not use the dentist and called me for the name of a Huggins trained dentist.

Now to the point I made earlier and why a root canal is the worst thing for a woman, Dr Huggins did extensive research over many decades and part of that was specifically on root canals.

He found that a very large percentage of women that died of breast cancer also had a root canal; I believe it was more than 90%. Now that's not a coincidence, if it had been 15 %or 20% then I suppose it could be written off as a coincidence but in excess of 90% then no, it's just too much.

I'll clarify what I mean here, this doesn't mean that if you're a woman and you have a root canal you'll get breast cancer; it means you have a greater chance of getting breast cancer if you have a root canal.

Similarly just because you smoke it doesn't mean you'll get lung cancer however there is a far greater chance of getting lung cancer if you smoke than if you don't.

So is there an alternative to root canals?, yes to get the same long term effects of course there is an alternative, try taking small doses of strychnine on a daily basis. Sorry for my flippancy, but the strychnine will devastate your body, slowly which is similar to what happens with root canals?

When the dentist does the root canal, he or she drills through the enamel and cleans out the dentin tubules of which there are more than 3 miles of these microscopic tubes. Then removes the pulp chamber, so the tooth is now dead, it's then filled with a wax called Gutta Percha which is heated. The tooth is sealed, now anything that is warm will cool over time. When the Gutta Percha cools, it shrinks causing little voids in the tooth, there are bacteria which were aerobic bacteria which require oxygen, but they mutate into anaerobic bacteria that can thrive in the absence of oxygen.

Some of those bacteria are more toxic than **botulism or tetanus.**

When the tooth is dead it creates other problems, the bacteria accumulating in the tooth is bad enough, however it gets worse, blood normally flows to the tooth to help move the nutrients to the living tooth. But it's dead so the blood doesn't provide the necessary nutrition anymore. The tooth attaches to the bone via something called a periodontal ligament, when the tooth originally grew in your mouth this ligament was formed. Six different types of strands form the ligament, there are thousands of them forming a shock absorber between the tooth and the bone. Three types grow down from the tooth and three types grow up from the bone intermeshing to form this hammock if you will.

So because it's dead there are anaerobic bacteria in the tooth and around the tooth in the periodontal ligament, so it's no wonder a large percentage of root canals are re done and often several times.

There is no such thing as a sterile root canal... it is very misleading when you are told it's a successful root canal. What is really meant is that it's an unsuccessful root canal, yes it's solid and it's not giving you pain at the moment but it is causing other problems it's just that you aren't aware of them yet.

When something is in your body that your body doesn't like, you experience problems, your immune system lets you know by way of a symptom. It's your body's way of telling you something isn't right. Something shouldn't be there, it's not natural and your body is trying to eliminate it. What do you do, you see a doctor or dentist and they give you a drug which mask's the symptom. Keeping this as simple and understandable as possible, there are little switches in your body that say…PAIN… the drug turns that switch off. The problem is still there but you have been told to adopt the ostrich attitude and bury your head in the sand.

As I mentioned earlier, a root canal is in the best interest of the dentist, not you. But you have pain in your mouth and quite often its excruciating pain. Now there might be a genuine case for removing the tooth, I know that doesn't sound like a good option but it has to be considered if the tooth is dead. However there may be an alternative and one that is very easy to do.

Now I know lots of people are going to read what I say now and just dismiss it without a second thought. Vitamin C is one of the most overlooked and underrated vitamins; I'm not talking about the standard dose recommended by the authority that appears to have no idea of its true value or concern for your health.

Now I'm not saying that this will cure the problem but I am telling you that Vitamin C will help. When you have bacteria in your blood, and there are various ways it might have got there. You might have had a fall and knocked the tooth loose. You might have eaten some foods that didn't agree with you or it might have been the fact you've been doing something wrong for your body for many years and your immune system has said **"enough",** the sign for this is pain. When bacteria gets into the blood it will manifest itself in a variety of ways, if this is in your mouth then the likelihood is that it will show itself as an abscess. This is just as likely to be a rash on your skin or an ache in a joint.

Firstly I'd make sure you have sodium ascorbate powder (Vit-C), there are numerous places you can get a decent sodium ascorbate from but my recommendations are:

Brunson product, 1 800 610 4848

Huggins Applied Healing, 1 866 948 4638

Either one is good, so this is how it's used.

¼ teaspoon in 2 oz's water then put ½ oz of the water into your mouth, lean your head to the side so the water and sodium ascorbate cover the tooth that is infected. Let it bathe in the water for 45 seconds then spit it out, don't flush it around your mouth just let it sit over the infected tooth. Repeat the process three more times until all the water is gone.

Repeat that process 6 times each day.

Do this for 7 days.

I can just hear some of you saying, "That's a pain in the butt, I'm not going to do that" well it's a very easy and cheap alternative to losing the tooth and certainly a lot less traumatic and painful than having a root canal.

VITAMIN C

Vitamin-C is probably the most overlooked and underrated vitamin, the reason for this is quite simple. It's cheap, very readily available, it works in a multitude of positive ways oh and the biggest reason is that Big Pharma can't make billions of dollars ripping off innocent people.

Now don't rush out and buy copious amounts of Vitamin C to throw down your throat, please read this chapter and have a better understanding of how this incredible vitamin can improve your life.

Taking vitamin-C orally in large doses will more than likely induce diarrhea, I personally take 10g's per day, I didn't just jump up to 10 grams, I started with 1g per day and did that for a few days then gradually increased the dose by 1g every few days until I was taking 10g's per day.

D.r Levy who I'll talk about in more detail recommends taking between 7-15g's per day, and Dr Huggins says that by taking just 3g's per day will mean it's unlikely you will ever have a cold or the flu again.

I'll start by telling you about this incredible man, Thomas E Levy, MD, JD. Wonderful combination, doctor and lawyer, now I think he has a very good understanding of what he can and can't say.

A product Dr Levy promotes very strongly is Lypo-Spheric Vit-C; this comes in small 1g packs. You might remember earlier I talked about small doses of Vit-C and how that's not very effective. Well this comes in a liposomal form, a gel that is absorbed in the small intestine so it has the same effect as 8.25 grams of regular vitamin C. You can get this product which I strongly recommend from Livon Labs..

1-866-790-2107

www.livonlabs.com

What Thomas E. Levy, MD, JD, says about Lypo-Spheric™ Vitamin C

"Comparing the bioavail-ability of all other oral vitamin C delivery with your oral liposomal delivery is like comparing a squirt gun to a fire hose. Not only am I convinced that the efficacy of Lypo-Spheric™ Vitamin C far surpasses any traditional oral vitamin C supplement, but my recent personal experience with it suggests that it may sometimes be better than IV injection."

So what are liposomes, exactly?

Liposome Articles Liposome-Encapsulated Products

Liposomes are belayed (double-layer), liquid-filled bubbles made from phospholipids. Over 50 years ago, researchers discovered that these spheres could be filled with therapeutic agents and used to protect and deliver these agents into the body and even into specific cells of the body.

The belayed structure of liposomes is nearly identical to the belayed construction of the cell membranes that surround each of the cells in the human body. This occurs because of the unique composition of phospholipids. The phosphate (source of "phospho" in phospholipid) head of phospholipids is hydrophilic — it loves water — whereas the fatty-acid tails (lipids) are hydrophobic — they hate water.

Liposome containing vitamin C. Currently liposome-encapsulation is the best oral way to deliver vitamin C known to man.

When phospholipids find themselves in a water-based solution, the hydrophobic tails quickly move to distance themselves from the liquid just like oil separates from vinegar. So, as all the tails turn inward and all the heads turn toward the liquid, they form a double-layered membrane with all the tails pointing toward one another and the heads facing the outside or the inside of the sphere that they have formed.

Now let's go back in time to the last century, the 1940's, Dr. Frederick Klenner, a general practitioner specializing in disease of the chest. A man was brought into the hospital with encephalitis which at that time was another of the incurable diseases.

The hospital basically said "there is nothing we can do for him, put him into the ward, he'll be dead in two days.

Dr. Klenner suggested that he could help him; you can imagine the response from the other doctors. Anyway Dr. Klenner gave him 5,000 mg of vitamin c intravenously three times each day for three days. On the fourth day he was discharged from hospital and on the fifth day he went back to work.

http://www.doctoryourself.com/klennerbio.html

Great information about Dr. Klenner and his work with polio patients.

CHOLESTEROL

I THINK THERE IS MORE MISINFORMATION about cholesterol than anything else, the average person has been duped and mislead into thinking that cholesterol is bad, it's actually a saint not a sinner.

There really isn't bad cholesterol; yes there are types of cholesterol but not just two as is often thought.

HDL is high density lipoproteins

LDL is low density lipoproteins

VLDL is very low density lipoproteins and they all have a place, they have a valid reason to be in the body.

The body manufactures around 60% of the cholesterol it needs to function, so you require the other 40% from foods.

As vegetables do not contain cholesterol your body needs to get it from an animal diet.

Cholesterol is the second biggest natural detoxifier in the body, Albumin being the biggest. So when you are exposed to toxins either through your diet or some other avenue the cholesterol sets about neutralizing them.

I suppose that it's fair to say that cholesterol is guilty by association, if you did a survey of the accidents in your local city you'd find that every time there was a vehicle accident, there was also an ambulance present. It would it be fair to suggest that the ambulance was the common denominator, but unfair to say that the ambulance was the guilty party when it came to vehicle accidents. No, the ambulance was there because of the accident and the same applies to cholesterol. As the second biggest natural detoxifier it rushes in to protect you and eliminate the toxins, but what happens is the medical profession see you have high cholesterol **in their opinion** and give you a statin drug.

The statin artificially lowers your cholesterol and enables the toxins to run riot, you suffer a heart attack or stroke and the doctor says," *I'm sorry it was just because of your high cholesterol, we prescribed an anticcholestrol medication but the cholesterol was too high and we couldn't get it down quick enough*".

This is a load of rubbish, cholesterol is there to help you, God didn't put us on this planet to commit suicide, he gave us all we need to survive and thrive, but sadly the greedy amongst us have provided lots of tasty appealing

treats. But those treats cause problems in our body, so we are told about options that supposedly help. They don't help really; they just put a band aid on the problem.

In the book Nutrition and Physical Degeneration written by Dr. Weston A Price, he found that as the volume of fats in the diet went down, the race degenerated, he said that the people with the best overall health around the world had about 40% fat in their diet. He monitored the cholesterol and triglyceride levels for almost twenty years and found that there is no relationship between the amount of fats in the diet and the serum level of fats.

Cholesterol makes up approximately 25% of the dry weight of the brain, and at least 23% of the cell membrane of the red blood cells, without this they wouldn't be able to flex and contort and get through the tiny capillaries resulting in local necrosis, in the brain this is known as a stroke.

I mentioned butter before as an essential ingredient to the diet, Dr. Huggins has recommended as much as a quarter pound of butter daily. The reason for this is that the intestinal tract is essentially a giant fat soluble membrane.

Nutrients appear to be absorbed better across a fat soluble when they are in conjunction with fats. Butter supplies this form of fat. Dr. Huggins noted that when overweight people change from margarine to butter they tend to lose weight very easily. The reason for this may be that the body is actually hungry for nutrients, so as the nutrients are absorbed via the mechanism of fat, the hunger desire is satisfied more easily. Another point to make here is that fats are fats and oils are oils, they are similar but not the same.

A very interesting and valid point to also make in regards to margarine, when you break down margarine into its cellular form you'll find it is **very similar to plastic...**

If you place an open tub of margarine in your garden and next to it place an open tub of butter, then leave them for a week You'll find all of the butter has gone but the margarine is still intact. Even insects know its bad and won't touch it.

When margarine was originally created it was as a fattening agent for turkeys, the turkeys wouldn't' touch it. The creators had spent millions and millions in development. When the turkeys ignored this costly fact the manufacturers had to do something, so they added a coloring agent to make it look more like butter and sold it for human consumption..

The HDL has a very influential role to play in protection against heart disease amongst other things; HDL is from the cholesterol fraction of the blood the LDL from the cholesterol and triglyceride fraction while the VLDL only from the triglyceride fraction. LDL and VLDL combine in the liver with Bilirubin to produce bile which is essential in metabolizing foods. When this isn't done correctly, food is not synthesized or absorbed correctly, resulting in gallstones in the liver and gallbladder.

Andreas Moritz PhD explains how gallstones are formed in the liver and gallbladder in his book listed below. I found it to be a very interesting book and was totally amazed to discover the prevalence of liver and gallbladder problems in America today. I had heard about people having an operation to have gallstones removed. I really had no idea that most people have gallstones but aren't aware of the problems yet. Moritz talks about not just having a gallstone or ten or twenty gallstones but how some people can have as many as 20,000 gallstones. Yes you read that correctly, 20,000 gallstones.

He details in his book how gallstones are formed and more importantly goes into great detail on how to remove them, ***without an operation.***

How this can be done from home relat*ively painlessly* over a six day period, this is a great book to read, I bought my copy as an e-book from Barnes and Noble for $9.95.

Back to cholesterol, statistically there are far more problems with having low cholesterol than high cholesterol, more people suffer from stroke when their cholesterol is below 160 mg% and more people die of cancer when their cholesterol is below 150 mg%.

Studies have shown other significant problems such as depression and leading to suicide. There are many cases of vandalism and hooliganism, fighting and bad behavior due to low cholesterol.

Two very well respected medical professionals on this subject are Thomas E Levy, MD, JD and Hal Huggins, MS, DDS, their work differs slightly in the correct level but both show proof that it should be higher than your traditional doctor is recommending in keeping your cholesterol below 175 mg%.

Huggins' grand mentor was Melvin Page DDS who suggests a level of 221 mg% while Levy talks about 240-250 mg%.

When I met Dr. Huggins in 2007 I had a blood test for the Huggins recovery program and was shocked to find my cholesterol was at 274 mg%. Doc suggested that I eat more eggs and butter to remedy that problem.

You can imagine the shocked look on my face at hearing this; however I followed his advice and ate 2 eggs and large amounts of butter each day. Two weeks later I had another blood test and was very pleasantly surprised to see my cholesterol was down to 238 mg%. Yes that happened in only two weeks, you have probably heard from your doctor that when your cholesterol is high you'll have to go on a statin drug and probably be on that medication for life.

One of my first questions to Dr. Huggins was "how do you raise your cholesterol if it's too low, he replied with "eat two eggs per day and a quarter pound of butter" I then asked "how do you lower it if it's too high" when he told me the same thing "eat two eggs and a quarter pound of butter" I was a little shocked to say the least.

Your body will find the natural, healthy level for cholesterol.

There is a wealth of information on this subject if you care to read the following books:

Optimal Nutrition for Optimal Health, Thomas E Levy, MD, JD

The Liver and Gallbladder miracle cleanse, Andreas Moritz, PhD

HIDDEN CONTAMINANTS

I KNOW THIS IS GOING TO upset a lot of people but it has to be said, the three worst foods you can put into your body are as follows:

Sugar, alcohol and caffeine, in that order.

All carbohydrates consumed will at some point be converted into sugar in the body; the average consumption of sugar worldwide is more than 43 lbs per person per year.

That isn't the case for Americans where sugar is consumed at a much higher level; in fact it's closer to 140 lbs per person per year.

The problem is that sugars will imbalance the chemistries of carbohydrate metabolism and it does this more dramatically than anything else.

Sugar affects the balance of calcium and phosphorus these two should have a ratio of 2 ½ to 1, an ideal balanced ration is 10 mg% to 4mg% of calcium to phosphorus.

When this balance is upset you may experience calculus on the teeth, cataracts in the eyes, kidney stones, gallstones, arthritis or arterial sclerosis. However, correcting this imbalance has shown a reversal in these problems.

A good alternative to sugar is not the sugar substitutes like Aspartame or high fructose corn syrup, but honey or agave nectar.

I'll mention this now before I forget; aspartame is probably in close to 9,000 food and drink products sold in America. Aspartame has been shown to mimic the detrimental effects of multiple sclerosis. It affects the pancreas negatively, believing it has to deal with sugar and addressing the insulin issue when in reality that isn't a problem so the pancreas is overworked. It's the "cry wolf" syndrome so when the pancreas is actually called into play it simply can't do its job properly.

Aspartame is converted into methanol, then into formic acid (fire ants inject formic acid when they bite) then into formaldehyde which as you know, is embalming fluid, not nice for the living body.

Alcohol, most populations around the world have alcohol built into their social life, in fact when a person doesn't drink alcohol he or she is often seen as a strange person.

I'll not go into depth on this subject because I believe most people already know of the detrimental effects alcohol can have on your liver and kidneys.

I think you all know that hard liquor is harder on your body than beer or wine, wine is probably the easiest for the body to assimilate and has less harmful effects on your chemistries. White wine is closer to the body's natural ph so is easier to deal with. I suppose if you are going to drink when you socialize then white wine would be considered more acceptable.

Caffeine, looking back on my time with Dr. Huggins I distinctly remember him talking more negatively about caffeine than anything else. In fact I remember him telling me that if caffeine disappeared off the face of the earth then probably 40% of physicians would be out of work.

One cup of coffee requires roughly 3 units of insulin to metabolize; a doctor had a relative with diabetes who was taking 18 units of insulin per day. He asked how much coffee he drank and was told about 6 cups per day. He put two and two together as in 6 cups of coffee each requiring 3 units of insulin equaling 18 units. He explained his understanding and suggested not drinking coffee as a way of eliminating the diabetes. He stopped drinking coffee but continued with the insulin which resulted in insulin shock. I'm not suggesting you take this action believing it will rid you of diabetes however it should be considered and discussed with your medical professional.

There are about 30 mgs of caffeine in the average candy bar (chocolate, you'll find about 125 mgs in a cup of coffee, however a regular Starbucks contains around 250 mgs and their Grande has approximately 550 mgs.

Starbucks also put other ingredients in their coffee (excitotoxins) which make you crave a "Starbucks" not just a coffee.

You'll also find caffeine in most tea's plus soft drinks; this can vary from as little as 34 mgs to more than 70 mgs.

TOOTH DECAY, AND THE REAL REASON IT HAPPENS

Some of the most in interesting reading I came across while working for Dr. Huggins was about Dr. Ralph Steinman while working at Loma Linda University in California regarding rats and tooth decay.

26 days in a rat's life is roughly equal to one human year, Dr Steinman published more than 70 articles on the systemic reaction of sugar in the body. There is a fluid flow through the tooth that is affected by sugar, the fluid flows naturally from the pulp chamber, through the dentin tubules then through the enamel. Sugar reverses this flow resulting in decay.

In one article he talked about rats that were fed through a tube, the first group was fed a sugar solution (62%) directly into their body bypassing the mouth. The rats developed

5.6 cavities. Bear in mind that the sugar water never came into contact with the teeth. The next group was fed soy milk and they developed 7.8 cavities, when they were fed homogenized milk it went up to 9.4 cavities.

This all sounds really bad but it gets worse because when they were fed chocolate milk it escalated to 21.8 cavities. This is because of the vanadium being blocked by the chocolate which in turn blocks the action of chromium which controls the glucose.

You could almost say that eating candy bars instead of drinking milk would cause fewer cavities in the teeth because a candy bar is less than 62% sugar. I'm not advocating this, just commenting on Dr. Steinman's work.

HEALTHY FATS

1. Pineapple (200 words)

PINEAPPLE IS A TROPICAL FRUIT that contains an enzyme called bromelain, which aids in digestion and reduces bloating. Bromelain helps break down proteins and promotes the absorption of nutrients, ensuring efficient digestion. Pineapple is also a natural diuretic, which can help reduce water retention and contribute to a flatter stomach. Enjoy fresh pineapple as a snack, in smoothies, or as a topping for salads.

2. Whole Grains (200 words)

Incorporating whole grains into your diet, such as oats, quinoa, and brown rice, can support a flat stomach. Whole grains are rich in fiber, which aids in digestion, prevents constipation, and reduces bloating. They also have a lower glycemic index compared to refined grains, which means they are digested more slowly, providing a steady release of energy and preventing spikes in blood sugar levels. Opt for whole grain bread, pasta, and cereals to maximize the benefits.

3. Green Tea (150 words)

Green tea is not only a refreshing beverage but also a great addition to a flat stomach diet. It contains antioxidants called catechins that help boost metabolism and promote fat oxidation. Green tea also has mild diuretic properties, which can help reduce water retention. Enjoy a cup of green tea in the morning or throughout the day as a healthy alternative to sugary drinks.

4. Lean Proteins (200 words)

Including lean proteins in your meals can aid in achieving a flat stomach. Lean protein sources, such as skinless chicken, turkey, fish, tofu, and legumes, provide essential amino acids while being low in fat. Protein takes longer to digest, increases satiety, and helps build and repair muscles. Additionally, protein-rich foods have a higher thermic effect, meaning they require more energy to digest, which can slightly boost metabolism.

5. Peppermint (150 words)

Peppermint has been used for centuries to soothe digestive discomfort and reduce bloating. It contains menthol, which helps relax the muscles of the gastrointestinal tract, promoting smooth digestion. Peppermint tea or adding fresh mint leaves to your water or salads are simple ways to incorporate this stomach-friendly herb into your diet.

Conclusion (100 words)

Incorporating foods that aid digestion, reduce bloating, and promote a healthy gut can play a significant role in achieving a flat stomach. Including avocados, Greek yogurt, ginger, leafy greens, cucumbers, pineapple, whole grains, green tea, lean proteins, and peppermint in your diet can provide numerous benefits. Remember to combine a healthy eating plan with regular exercise and lifestyle habits to optimize your results. As always, consult with a healthcare professional or registered dietitian for personalized advice that suits your individual needs and goals. Embrace a nourishing and balanced diet, and enjoy the journey towards a flatter and healthier abdomen.

Summary

This book contains valuable information for the everyday person, during my three and a half years working for Dr. Huggins; I talked with more than 17,000 people. It never failed to amaze me how little most people knew. This isn't a slight on the public, more an observation of how those in the medical profession and the media have brainwashed the masses. I don't really know if the doctors actually believe they are helping a patient by giving them a drug to address the symptom rather than the cause, or the dentist who places an amalgam filling or root canal.

At this time the pharmaceutical industry holds the balance of power, they can spend millions of dollars through lobbyist in DC and billions on advertising so the government may see them as helping the economy and keeping people in jobs.

If I can play a small part in educating people and saving one life then my book is a success.

My website is full of more very helpful information.

www.ratherbehealthy.com

HUGGINS TRAINED DENTISTS

Alabama.

Dr. Ada Frazier	256 828 1599,	Meridianville, AL
Dr. Dayton Hart	251 943 2471,	Foley, AL

Arizona

Dr. Nicholas Hart	480 948 0560,	Scottsdale, AZ
Dr. Brett Benson	480 414 8115,	Chandler, AZ

California

Dr. Dian Olah	310 858 9212,	Beverly Hills, CA
Dr. Pearl Zadeh	818 716 6722,	Woodland Hills, CA
Dr. P Vernon Erwin	818 246 1748,	Glendale, CA
Dr. Wayne Wu	949 788 0088,	Irvine, CA
Dr. Robert Garabedian	559 229 6553,	Fresno, CA
Dr. David Partrite	925 837 3101,	Danville, CA
Dr. Andrew Zakarian	619 296 6899,	San Diego, CA

Colorado

Dr. John Augspurger	719 597 5900,	Colorado Springs, CO
Dr. David Winn	719 260 9000,	Colorado Springs, CO
Dr. John Rothchild	970 382 7780,	Durango, CO
Dr. Dale Strietzel	970 247 3303,	Durango, CO
Dr. Denise Vandewalle	719 589 4771,	Alamosa, CO

Florida

Dr. Hank Barreto	305 271 8321,	Coral Gables, FL
Dr. Huguette, Duteau	727 323 8118,	St Pete, FL
Dr. Fredda Rosenbaum	305 933 3350,	Aventura, FL

Hawaii

Dr. Barkley Bastian	808 572 9461,	Makawao, HI

Idaho

Dr. Vernon Gaffner	208 524 2034,	Idaho Falls, ID
Dr. Russ Misner	208 476 5437,	Pocatello, ID

Illinois

Dr. Paul Gallo	815 741 2752,	Joliet, IL
Dr. Terry Cavanaugh	630 986 5150,	Hinsdale, IL
Dr. Carl Henley	630 357 9393,	Naperville, IL
Dr. Kathleen Minaghan	708 848 4488,	Oak Park, IL
Dr. Diane Meyer	630 968 5567,	Downers Grove, IL

Massachusetts

Dr. Robert Evans	978 449 9919,	Groton, MA

Maryland

Dr. Eugene Sambataro	410 964 3118,	Ellicott City (Baltimore) MD

Michigan
Dr. Kevin Flood   616 974 4990,   Grand Rapids, MI

Missouri
Dr. Michael Rehme   314 997 2550,   St Louis, MO

New Jersey
Dr. Elizabeth Piela   732 280 9700,   Belmar, NJ

New York
Dr. Israel Brenner   631 271 1770,   Huntington, NY

North Carolina
Dr. Michael Willock   919 942 2154,   Chapel Hills, NC
Dr. Bill Virtue   336 679 2034,   Winston Salem, NC

Ohio
Dr. Greg Buerschen   937 241 2154,   Dayton, OH
Dr. John Johnson   614 775 9300,   New Albany, OH
Dr. John Johnson   740 427 7122,   Mount Vernon, OH

Oregon
Dr. Anne Herff Meyer   541 265 8551,   Newport, OR

Pennsylvania
Dr. Blanche Grube   570 343 1500,   Scranton, PA

Texas
Dr. Stuart Nunnally   830 693 3646,   Marble Falls, TX
Dr. Dickie Stanley   830 693 0748,   Marble Falls, TX
Dr. Marilyn Jones   713 785 7767,   Houston, TX
Dr. Bill Glaros   281 440 1190,   Houston, TX
Dr. Daniel Strader   214 363 7777,   Dallas, TX

Utah

Dr. Wendell Robertson   801 798 6023,   Spanish Fork, UT

Virginia

Dr. Robert Johnson   703 246 9355,   Fairfax, VI

Washington

Dr. Tom Seal   425 823 9000,   Kirkland, WA

Wisconsin

Dr. Ingo Mahn   262 691 4555,   Pewaukee, WI

Mexico

Dr. Ezekiel Lagos   1 877 356 0056,   Tijuana, MX

Canada

Dr. Ewa Tobin   705 458 0775,   Thornton, ON

Dr. Dana Colson   416 482 2133,   Toronto, ON

Dr. Hans Schwartz   905 780 0083,   Stouffville, ON

England

Dr. Igsaan Khan   0117 953 8383   Bristol, UK

Taiwan

Dr. Janet (Poo Jern Wong)   Taipei, Taiwan

Australia

Dr. Andrew Taylor   2 6687 2552,   Newrybar, NSW

Dr. Frank Depczynski   2 6752 2775.   Moree, NSW

Dr. Eric Davis   7 3284 5755   Margate Beach, QLD

GLOSSARY OF BOOKS

It's all in your head... Hal A Huggins, DDS, MS

Solving the MS mystery... Hal A Huggins, DDS, MS

It's right under your nose... Hal A Huggins, DDS, MS

Integrity VS. Intimidation...Hal A Huggins, DDS, MS

Uninformed Consent... Hal Huggins MS, DDS and Thomas E Levy, MD, JD

Optimal Nutrition for Optimal Health... Thomas E Levy, MD, JD

Stop America's #1 Killer...Thomas E Levy, MD, JD

Curing the incurable...Thomas E Levy, MD, JD

Roots of disease..Robert Kulacz DDS and Thomas E Levy, MD, JD

The Liver and Gallbladder miracle cleanse, Andreas Moritz, PhD

ABOUT THE AUTHOR

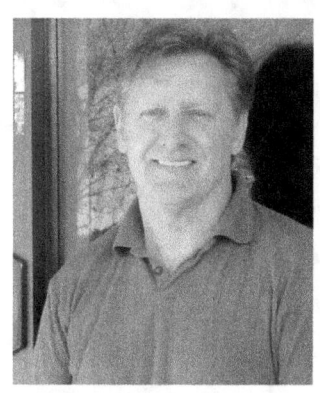

Stefan Cairns was born in Liverpool, England in 1955, he has participated in many sporting activities, some of which may be perceived as extreme sports.

Skydiving was a significant part of his life for many years, in fact Stefan has done almost 1,000 skydives and was part of the largest relative work formation in England in 1989.

The 60 way was actually in the Guinness Book of Records between 1989 and 1997.

He was also a hang glider pilot, scuba diver, rock climber, mountain biker and a pilot, these activities were all brought to a halt when Stefan was diagnosed with multiple sclerosis in 2004.

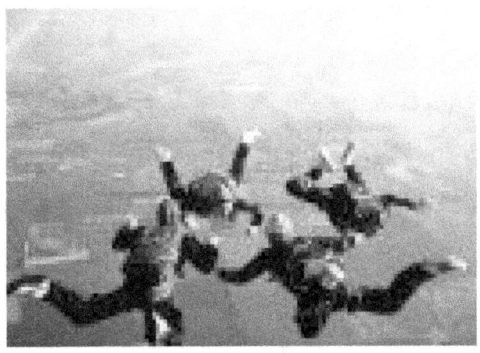